Copyright © 2022 by An~~~ ~~~~~~

Table of Contents

NEUROPATHY DIET

Diabetes, a disease characterized by blood glucose (sugar) levels that are too high (called hyperglycemia), is the most common cause of neuropathy.

People with diabetic neuropathy should eat to maintain the blood glucose levels their doctors recommend, which includes limiting sweets, beverages with added sugar, and large portions of foods that are high in starches or carbohydrates. Instead, opt for a diet that leans toward portion-controlled high-fiber/whole grains, vegetables, fruits, low- or nonfat dairy, and lean proteins like boneless, skinless chicken breast, fish, and turkey.

NEUROPATHY DIET RECIPES

1. Louisiana Gumbo

Total Time: 50 mins

Servings:4

Ingredients

- ¼ cup all-purpose flour
- 1 tablespoon canola oil
- 1 onion, chopped
- 1 large green bell pepper, diced
- 1 stalk celery, minced
- 4 cloves garlic, minced
- 4 cups reduced-sodium chicken broth
- 1 14-ounce can whole tomatoes, drained and chopped
- 10 okra pods, trimmed and cut into 1/2-inch-long pieces (1 cup)
- ½ teaspoon freshly ground pepper
- ¼ teaspoon dried thyme
- ¼ teaspoon dried oregano
- ⅛ teaspoon cayenne pepper

- 1 bay leaf
- ½ cup long-grain white rice
- 6 ounces medium shrimp, peeled and deveined
- 4 ounces boneless, skinless chicken breast, or thigh meat, trimmed and cut into 1/2-inch pieces
- 2 ounces andouille or kielbasa sausage, thinly sliced
- Salt, to taste
- Hot sauce, to taste

Directions

1. Heat a heavy cast-iron skillet over medium heat. Add flour and cook, stirring constantly with a wooden spoon, until the flour turns a deep golden color, 7 to 10 minutes. Transfer the flour to a plate and let cool. (There will be a strong aroma similar to burnt toast. Be careful not to let the flour burn; reduce the heat if flour seems to be browning too quickly.) Alternately, toast the flour in a pie plate in a 400 degrees F oven for 20 minutes.

2. Heat oil in a heavy stockpot over medium heat. Add onion, bell pepper, celery and garlic; sauté

until the onions are lightly browned, about 7 minutes. Stir in the toasted flour. Gradually stir in broth and bring to a simmer, stirring. Add tomatoes, okra, pepper, thyme, oregano, cayenne and bay leaf. Cover and cook for 15 minutes. Stir in rice and cook, covered, for 15 minutes longer.

3. Add shrimp, chicken and sausage; simmer until the shrimp is opaque inside, the chicken is no longer pink and the rice is tender, about 5 minutes longer. Discard the bay leaf and season with salt. Ladle into bowls and serve with hot sauce.

2. Asparagus, Lima Bean & Almond Pasta

Ingredients

- 3 tablespoons almonds, sliced
- 1 tablespoon sea salt, for the pasta water
- 8 ounces whole wheat rotini or penne pasta
- 1 pound green asparagus, trimmed and cut into 1-inch pieces
- 1 cup frozen baby lima beans
- 3 tablespoons olive oil
- 2 cloves garlic, smashed, peeled and thinly sliced
- 1 dried pepper pod, de-seeded (optional)
- 3 tablespoons Italian parsley, chopped
- 1 tablespoon Parmigiano Reggiano cheese, grated (optional)
- Sea salt and black pepper to taste

Directions

1. Toast the sliced almonds in a heavy- wide pan until they are just turning golden. Transfer to a bowl and set aside.
2. Bring salted water to a boil in a large pot. Add pasta to the boiling water and continue to boil for

7 minutes, or 3 minutes less than package instructions. Add the asparagus and frozen lima beans to the boiling pasta and cook for 2 minutes. Reserve 1 cup of pasta water, then drain the pasta and vegetables -- they should be a little undercooked.

3. Meanwhile, in a deep pan or wok, heat olive oil over medium-high heat. Once the oil is hot, add the garlic and chili pepper, if using. Continue cooking until the garlic is light gold, about 3 minutes. Do not let the garlic burn.

4. Add the parsley to the pan and stir-fry for 1 minute. Add ¼ cup of pasta water to the pan and bring to a simmer. Add the almonds, and turn the heat down to medium. If the pan gets dry, add more pasta water, a little at a time.

5. Add the drained pasta, asparagus, and lima beans to the pan. Stir well, and add in the remaining pasta water, stirring continuously and allowing to reduce. Add the grated cheese and a grind or two of black pepper. Mix well and cook for another minute. Taste for seasonings then serve.

3. Omega-3-Packed Avocado Toast

Ingredients

- ½ ripe Hass avocado
- 2 slices whole-grain toast or good white sourdough toast
- Salt and pepper, to taste
- A drizzle of honey, agave, or olive oil (optional)
- 2 tablespoons sunflower seeds (optional)
- 2 teaspoons ground flaxseed (optional)
- 2 teaspoons chia seed (optional)
- 1 cup arugula, tightly packed

Directions

1. Scoop out the avocado flesh and spread it onto the toast by mashing it with the back of a fork. Sprinkle salt, pepper, and a drizzle of honey, if using.
2. Add seeds, if using, and top with arugula.

4. Bananas Baked in Coconut

Ingredients

- 6 ripe bananas
- 3 tablespoons melted coconut oil
- Freshly grated nutmeg to taste (optional)
- Greek yogurt for serving (optional)

Directions

1. Preheat the oven to 425 degrees. Line a baking tray with parchment paper. Set aside.
2. Pour the melted coconut oil into a shallow bowl or plate.
3. Peel the bananas, cutting off the tops and bottoms. Carefully cut them in half lengthwise. Roll them around in the oil until well coated and lay them, cut side down, onto the prepared baking sheet. Brush them with any remaining oil and grate a little nutmeg over them, if using.
4. Bake for 20 minutes on a high shelf. Turn the bananas carefully with a spatula -- don't break them -- and return them to the oven for another 10 minutes or so until they're golden with

caramelized edges. Carefully lift them from the tray and serve warm with a dollop of Greek yogurt.

5. Basic Poached Salmon
Ingredients

- 1 small onion, peeled and halved
- 4 whole cloves
- 1 inch slice of lemon peel
- 1 teaspoon whole black peppercorns
- 1 bay leaf
- 1 large carrot, thickly sliced
- 1 stick celery or 2 fennel branches, stripped of their leaves
- 1 teaspoon sea salt, or to taste
- 4 to 6 cups water
- 1 fillet of salmon (about 2 ½ pounds), skin on, bones removed, rinsed and patted dry

Directions

1. Stick the onion halves with the cloves, 2 per half. In a wide sauté pan add the lemon peel, peppercorns, bay leaf, sea salt and all the vegetables, plus enough water to just cover it all. Bring the mixture to a boil over medium-high heat. Cover, turn the heat down to low and

simmer until the vegetables begin to soften, about 20 minutes.

2. When the vegetables are cooked, bring the stock back to a gentle boil. Place the salmon skin-side down on top of the vegetables and cover the pan tightly with a lid or foil so that no steam can escape. Turn off the heat.

3. Move the pan to the back of the stove and leave the salmon to steam for 8-10 minutes per inch of thickness, or until it has completely cooled. If you are poaching a whole fillet, check after 15 minutes. Don't open the lid before then -- you will let out all the steam and stop the cooking.

4. When the salmon is ready, gently lift it off the vegetables skin-side down with a plate or cutting board large enough to hold it in one piece. Take care not to break it. Cover with a 2nd disposable board or a plate big enough to cover it. Carefully flip it over. Remove the skin. Cover with the plate again. Carefully flip it back to right side up. Slide it onto a serving plate, trim, decorate and serve. Try it with our Roasted Broccoli recipe, or with our Vegetable "Dirty Rice".

6. Braised Collard Greens

Ingredients

- 1 medium onion, chopped
- 1 tablespoon olive oil
- 2 bunches collard greens, leaves chopped, stems discarded
- Salt, to taste
- 1 teaspoon smoked paprika
- 2 teaspoons cider or white wine vinegar
- 2 cups chicken or vegetable stock

Directions

1. Heat the olive oil in a medium pot over medium-high heat. Add the onions and cook, stirring occasionally until translucent, about 5-8 minutes.
2. Add the collard greens, sprinkle some salt over them, cover and let steam for 5 minutes.
3. Add the paprika, cook or a minute, then add the cider vinegar, and stock. Cover and cook over low heat for 40 minutes or until very tender.

7. Breakfast Couscous

Ingredients

- 1¼ cup milk or almond milk
- ½ cup whole wheat couscous
- ½ teaspoon cinnamon
- ½ teaspoon ground ginger
- 2 cardamom pods or cloves
- 2 tablespoons chopped almonds
- 2 tablespoons chopped prunes
- 2 tablespoons golden raisins

Directions

1. In a microwave proof bowl, combine the milk with cinnamon, honey, ground ginger, and cardamom. Cover and microwave for 2 minutes, until the milk is very warm and steaming.
2. Remove the bowl from the microwave. Remove the cardamom pods and stir in the couscous. Cover and let sit for 10 minutes, or until the milk has been absorbed. Stir in chopped almonds and dried fruit and enjoy warm.

8. Collard Greens & White Bean Soup
Ingredients

- 1 large bunch young collard greens or 2 small ones, leaves stripped from the hard stems and washed
- 1 to 2 tablespoons olive oil
- 1 sprig plus 1 teaspoon of fresh rosemary, leaves stripped and chopped
- 1 medium onion, finely diced
- 1 large carrot, cut into a small dice
- 1 medium Yukon Gold potato or other waxy potato, cut into a small dice
- 1 clove garlic, chopped
- 2 cups cooked baby lima or other white beans (cannellini or Great Northern), plus their broth or 1 (14-ounce) can, drained and rinsed well, plus ½ cup fresh water
- 2¼ quarts (9 cups) low-sodium vegetable or chicken stock, or water
- 1 tablespoon chopped flat-leaf parsley

Directions

1. Pull the leaves from their stems. Cut the leaves into bite-sized pieces. Set aside.

2. In a large Dutch oven, heat the oil over a medium-high flame until it starts to ripple. Add the rosemary. Let it sizzle for a moment, then add the onion, carrot, and potato. Mix well.

3. Turn the heat down to medium-low. Cover and sweat the vegetables for 8-10 minutes or until they are soft and the onion is slightly golden. Stir every so often to prevent sticking or burning.

4. Turn the heat up to medium high. Add the chopped garlic. Stir and cook for another 2 minutes until you start to smell its aroma. Add the collard greens and stir-fry until they start to wilt and soften.

5. Add the stock and beans, plus their liquid if home-cooked. The beans and vegetables should be well covered with liquid but not drowned. Add a little extra water if needed. Bring the soup to a boil. Partially cover and turn the heat down to

low. Simmer, stirring from time to time, for 20-25 minutes or until the greens are very tender.

6. Adjust seasoning, then cook 5 minutes more. Mash some of the beans against the sides of the pan to thicken the soup slightly. Stir in the chopped parsley and remaining rosemary. Cook 1 minute, then turn off the heat. Let the soup sit, covered, for 5 minutes. Serve drizzled with a little olive oil, if desired.

9. Egg Noodles in Broth

Ingredients

- 6 cups homemade Chicken Stock or Basic Vegetable Stock
- 16 oz of egg nest pasta
- 4 cups of baby spinach
- Parmesan cheese (optional)

Directions

1. Bring the broth to a boil. Break the pasta into the broth and cook until just tender. Break up the pasta with a kitchen knife if you want the noodles shorter.
2. Stir in the spinach, and cook for 2 more minutes. Serve with a little Parmesan cheese, if desired.

10. Fennel & Tomato Gratin

Ingredients

- 5 medium fennel bulbs, stalks removed
- 1 cup homemade breadcrumbs, or to taste
- ¾ cup finely grated Parmesan cheese
- Black pepper, to taste, Freshly ground
- 2 tablespoons olive oil
- For the Quick Tomato Sauce,
- 2 tablespoons olive oil
- 1 1/2 pounds ripe plum tomatoes (about 6-8), coarsely choppe
- 1 to 2 cloves garlic, smashed and thinly sliced lengthwise
- 1 small dried red pepper, seeds removed (optional)
- 1/2 teaspoon salt or to taste
- 1 tablespoons, freshly grated Parmesan cheese (optional)

Directions

1. Preheat the oven to 350 degrees F. Prepare the quick tomato sauce as outlined here.

2. Halve the fennel bulbs and parboil in salted water for about 10 minutes or until they are just soft and slightly translucent looking. Drain. Cut into quarters. If the bulbs are very large, cut each half into 3 pieces. Set aside.

3. Toss the breadcrumbs and the cheese together in a bowl. Set aside.

4. Bring the Quick Tomato Sauce to a boil over a medium high flame in a wide sauté pan. Lower the heat to medium and simmer until the sauce has thickened, about 10 to 15 minutes. Set aside.

5. Spread a thin layer of tomato sauce on the bottom of a shallow gratin dish, about â..." cup. Place the fennel cut sides down on top of the sauce in a tight single layer. Pour the rest of the sauce over them and spread evenly.

6. Sprinkle the fennel with the breadcrumb mixture until you have a generous crust. Drizzle with the olive oil and bake for 30 minutes covered with foil, then 10 minutes uncovered, or until the breadcrumbs are golden.

11. Healthy Fruity Oatmeal
Ingredients

- 1 ⅓ cups rolled oats (⅓ cup dry for 1 serving)
- 2 ⅔ cup water (⅔ cup water for ⅓ cup oatmeal)
- Generous pinch sea salt
- 1 tablespoon golden raisins
- 1 tablespoon dried cranberries
- ½ teaspoon cinnamon (optional)
- 2 apples (try tart Granny Smiths or Braeburns)
- 2 tablespoons almonds, sliced, dry toasted
- 2 bananas, thinly sliced
- Milk of your choice, or yogurt to taste

Directions

1. Mix the oats, water, salt, raisins, cranberries, and cinnamon in a pan. Bring to a boil, stir well and then lower the heat to a low simmer. Cook, covered, for about 10 minutes, stirring the oatmeal from time to time so that it doesn"t stick.

2. While the oatmeal is cooking, grate the apple using the coarsest bore. When the oatmeal has cooked, stir in the grated apple until it is well

mixed. Cover and turn the heat off. Leave the oatmeal for 5 minutes to steam.

3. Serve sprinkled with almonds and sliced bananas, and with milk or yogurt on the side.

12. Honeyed Miso Peanut Butter Spread

Ingredients

- ½ cup plus 2 tablespoons smooth all natural peanut butter
- ¼ cup white miso paste
- 1 tablespoon honey
- 1 tablespoon water

Directions

1. In a medium bowl, beat the peanut butter, miso paste, honey, and water together until they are completely blended.
2. If you want a softer or a runnier consistency, gradually add more water a teaspoon at a time until it"s how you want it.

13. Amazing Green Sauce

Ingredients

- 3 bunches of Lacinato kale, leaves stripped
- 6 cloves of garlic, smashed and skinned
- 1 teaspoon sea salt, or to taste
- ¼ cup extra virgin olive oil
- Freshly grated nutmeg, to taste

Directions

1. Put the kale and the whole garlic cloves into a large non-reactive pan with a lid. Add salt and just enough water to cover. Bring to a boil, then cover and simmer until the leaves are tender, about 15 – 20 minutes. Reserve a cup of the cooking water then drain.

2. Blend the cooked kale and garlic into a blender with olive oil, nutmeg, and ¼ cup of the reserved broth. Add more of the reserved water, a little at a time, if the sauce seems too stiff. The sauce should be very thick but pourable. Adjust seasoning and serve tossed with a short whole wheat pasta and freshly grated parmesan.

Ingredients

- ⅔ cup water
- Salt, to taste
- 1 dark green scallion stem
- 2 inch piece of lemon peel
- ¾ cup fresh or frozen peas
- ¾ cup chopped baby spinach
- 1 cup regular or whole wheat couscous (See Ann's Tips if you're on a Bland diet)
- 2 tablespoons chopped scallions, white and light green parts only (See Ann's Tips if you're on a Bland diet)
- Black pepper, to taste
- 4 Poached Eggs

Directions

1. In a medium stockpot, bring the water, salt and scallion stem to a boil.

2. Add the peas and baby spinach and continue to boil for 2 minutes. Turn off the heat, then stir in the couscous. Cover and let sit for 5 minutes.

3. Add the black pepper and chopped scallions if using and fluff the couscous with a fork. Taste for seasoning. Serve topped with a poached egg.

15. Peanut Butter Banana Oat Shake

Ingredients

- ¼ cup rolled oats
- ¼ cup water
- 1 cup milk
- 1 large ripe banana, peeled and cut into thirds
- 1 to 2 tablespoons unsweetened and unsalted peanut butter, or almond butter
- 2 teaspoons honey, or to taste
- ¼ to ½ teaspoon freshly ground nutmeg
- 2 ice cubes (optional)

Directions

1. In the microwave safe bowl combine the oatmeal and water. Microwave for 1 minute on high, or cook the oats in a small saucepan until the water has been absorbed. Set aside and let cool.

2. In a blender combine the oatmeal, milk, banana, peanut butter, honey, nutmeg, and ice cubes, if using. Blend until smooth. Best if served right away.

16. Provencal Tomato Soup
Ingredients

- 2 tablespoons olive oil
- 1 small onion, chopped
- 3 bay leaves
- Pinch of cayenne
- ¼ teaspoon brown sugar
- 2 pounds tomatoes, diced or 1 (28-ounce) can of chopped tomatoes
- 6 to 8 cloves of garlic, smashed and peeled
- 1 quart low-sodium stock or water
- ¼ cups pearl barley
- Parmesan rind (optional)
- Sea salt, to taste
- Fresh basil

Directions

1. Heat the oil over medium-high heat in a wide, heavy-bottomed pan. Add the onion and cook for a minute. Turn the heat to medium, add the bay leaves and sweat the onion until it starts to soften,

about 8 minutes. It shouldn't color, so stir from time to time to prevent it sticking and burning.

2. Turn the heat up to medium-high. Add the cayenne pepper, sugar and cook for a minute, then add the tomatoes and garlic. Cook, stirring until the tomatoes take on an orangey hue and have reduced a little.

3. Add the pearl barley, Parmesan rind, if using, and the stock, plus salt to taste. Bring to a simmer, lower the heat and cover. Cook until the barley is tender enough to smash with a spoon against the side of the pan, about 40 minutes. If substituting Arborio rice, it will take about half the amount of time to cook.

4. Let the soup sit for a few minutes. Remove the bay leaves and blend thoroughly, in batches, using either a wand blender or a freestanding one. Return to the pot, check the seasoning and add a grind or two of black pepper. Serve as is or with a few torn basil leaves or a little pesto stirred into it.

17. Pumpkin Miso Soup

Ingredients

- 1 small kabocha pumpkin, washed, halved, and seeds scraped out
- 2 tablespoon grape seed or canola oil
- 1 large Spanish onion, thinly sliced
- 8 to 10 cups low-sodium stock or water
- 2 to 3 tablespoons yellow miso paste (miso shiro), or to taste
- Sea salt and black pepper, to taste
- Soy sauce (optional)

Directions

1. With a peeler, take off little patches of skin all over the pumpkin halves until they look polka dotted. This is purely decorative and can be left out if you don't have time. Cut the halves into a ½-inch dice. Set aside.

2. Heat the oil in a large soup pot over a medium-high flame. When it ripples, add the onion and sauté, stirring until the onion starts to soften and turn transparent. Add the pumpkin cubes,

sprinkle with a little sea salt, mix well and cover. Turn the heat down to medium low and sweat the vegetables for about 10 minutes or until the pumpkin has started to soften and the onion is soft. The onion should not brown, so stir the pot occasionally to make sure it doesn't stick.

3. Add enough stock to the pot to cover the vegetables plus 1 inch. Raise the heat and bring to a boil. Cover, turn the heat to low, and simmer until the pumpkin is soft but not mushy, about 10 minutes. Do not overcook! While the soup is cooking, measure the miso into a bowl. Using a small balloon whisk or a fork, gradually whisk in ½ cup of warm stock or cool water until you have a thin-ish, creamy-looking liquid with no lumps.

4. When the pumpkin is tender, add a grind or two of black pepper, turn off the heat. Add the miso cream little by little, stirring gently to mix. Taste as you go until you know how much you like. Miso is richly salty, so you do not want too much in the soup. Check for seasoning. Serve immediately.

18. Green Kale Smoothie
Ingredients

- 3 leaves of kale, washed and chopped
- ¼ cup parsley sprigs
- Half of 1 medium apple, cored and cut into chunks
- ⅔ cup fresh or frozen mango, chopped
- 1 teaspoon fresh lemon juice
- ¾ cup cold water, or more if needed
- 2 ice cubes (optional)

Directions

1. Combine all ingredients in a blender and blend until smooth. If you are using fresh mangos, we recommend adding in the ice cubes. Best if served immediately.For more cancer-fighting treats, check out our Kale Recipes Slideshow!

19. Goat Cheese, Onion, Spinach & Lemon Pizza

Ingredients

- 1 teaspoon olive oil
- 1 clove garlic, smashed
- 2 cups packed baby spinach, washed
- 1 tablespoon panko or cornmeal
- 1 whole wheat pizza dough or refrigerated or frozen pizza crust
- ½ cup storebought tomato sauce or our Quick Tomato Sauce
- ¾ cup goat cheese
- ½ small onion, halved and thinly sliced
- ½ cup cherry tomatoes or grape tomatoes, halved
- 1 tablespoon olive oil
- Salt and pepper, to taste
- ½ a lemon, zested

Directions

1. Preheat the oven to 500 degrees F. Put 2 baking trays into the oven, or pizza stone if available.
2. In a medium sauté pan, over medium-high heat, add the 1 teaspoon of olive oil and clove of garlic.

Cook until the garlic starts to brown and become fragrant. Remove the garlic and add the baby spinach along with 1 tablespoon of water. Let sit for 1 minute and then stir. Once the spinach has wilted, remove from pan and let drain. Once cool enough, squeeze out excess liquid.

3. Sprinkle panko or cornmeal onto a large sheet of parchment paper. Roll out the dough onto the parchment paper; press out dough into a 12x8-inch rectangle or to fit your pizza stone. Split into two balls if necessary.

4. Spread the tomato sauce evenly onto the dough. Dot the pizza with the goat cheese and top it with the drained spinach, onions, and grape tomatoes, cut sides up. Drizzle with olive oil and sprinkle with a little salt and pepper.

5. Using the parchment paper, slip the pizza onto the heated baking trays or pizza stone. Bake in the oven on the lowest rack for 10-15 minutes, or until the crust is golden and the cheese looks melted.

6. Using the parchment paper, slip the pizza onto a cutting board. Sprinkle with the lemon zest and cut into slices.

20. Mango Granita

Ingredients

- 4 Champagne mangoes or 2 Tommy Atkin mangoes
- ¼ cup fine brown sugar (Florida Crystals), or to taste
- ½ a lemon, juiced

Directions

1. Remove the pit from the mango by cutting down each side of it through the stem end. Scoop out the flesh and put it into the blender. Trim any good mango from around the pit and add it to the rest. Add the sugar and lemon juice.
2. Blend all the ingredients together and pour into a glass or Pyrex bowl. Put into the freezer.
3. Check the bowl every 20 minutes or so to scrape the ice crystals off the sides of the bowl until you end up with a fluffy snowy consistency.

21. Chocolate Granita

Ingredients

- 2 cups water
- ½ cup sugar, or to taste
- ⅔ cup 100% cocoa powder (unsweetened)
- 1 teaspoon vanilla extract
- 3 ounces semi-sweet chocolate

Directions

1. In a medium saucepan combine the water, sugar, and cocoa powder. Whisk until smooth. Heat over medium-low heat. Once simmering, whisk in the vanilla extract and chocolate. Whisk until the chocolate has melted and is smooth. Taste for sweetness.

2. Transfer to a 9 x 9 x 2-inch glass baking pan. Leave to cool to room temperature then put in the freezer. After about 45 minutes, with a fork, scrape to form a flaky texture. Continue to scrape the surface every 30 minutes until fluffy and snow-like. Serve immediately or keep in an

airtight container in the freezer, scraping every so often to keep a light texture.

22. Coconut Granita
Ingredients

- 1¼ cups coconut milk
- ¾ cup cold water
- ¼ cup unsweetened toasted coconut flakes
- ½ teaspoon lime zest
- Juice from 1 lime
- 3 tablespoons to ¼ cup sugar, to taste

Directions

1. Mix all the ingredients together until well blended. Taste for sweetness.
2. Pour into a 9 x 9 x 2-inch glass baking pan and put into the freezer. After 30 minutes, with a fork scrape to form flaky texture. Continue to scrape the surface every 30 minutes until you have a fluffy snowy consistency. Serve or keep in an airtight container in the freezer, scraping every so often to keep a light texture.

23. Coffee Granita

Ingredients

- 2 cups freshly brewed strong coffee
- ½ teaspoon vanilla extract
- 3 to 4 tablespoons brown sugar or to taste, or ⅛ cup agave nectar

Directions

1. Blend all the ingredients together – if using sugar make sure it has melted into the coffee. Pour into a pyrex bowl and let it cool. Put in the freezer.
2. Check the bowl every 20 minutes or so, scraping the ice crystals off the sides of the bowl until you end up with a sorbet of a fluffy snowy consistency – about 2 hours.

24. Concord Grape Granita

Ingredients

- 2 cups Concord grapes, washed and stemmed
- 3 tablespoons of sugar (or to taste)
- Water, to cover
- 1 teaspoon lemon juice

Directions

1. Put the grapes into a small saucepan and cover with water. Add the sugar and bring to a boil. Turn the heat down to a simmer and cover. Cook for 20 - 30 minutes or until the skins are soft and the liquid syrupy. Add the lemon juice and cook 5 minutes more.

2. Press the fruit and syrup through a medium sieve into a ceramic bowl and let cool. Discard the seeds and any of the few tough skins that may be left behind in the sieve.

3. When the liquid is cool, put into the freezer. Every 15 to 20 minutes or so, scrape the icy crystals that form on the sides into the liquid. Keep doing this until the bowl is completely full of snowy textured

crystals. Serve immediately or leave in the freezer until you are ready. If the granita hardens, fluff it up again with a fork.

25. Peach Sweet Tea Granita
Ingredients

- 1 black tea bag (English Breakfast or Darjeeling)
- ¾ cup hot water
- 1 small ripe peach, peeled and diced
- 1 tablespoon lemon juice
- ¼ cup cold water
- 1 to 2 tablespoons sugar, to taste

Directions

1. Steep the tea bag with the hot water for 3 minutes. Discard the tea bag.
2. Puree the hot tea with the diced peaches until smooth. Stir in the lemon juice and sugar until the sugar is dissolved. Add the cold water. Taste for sweetness. Pour into a 9- by 9-inch baking pan. Cover and put into the freezer.
3. After 1 hour, using a fork, scrape the frozen top layer. Scrape and break any chunks into pieces. Continue to scrape every 15 to 20 minutes until the granita has a fluffy, snowy consistency –

about 2 hours. Eat immediately or keep for 3 days in the freezer, scraping every so often.

26. Blueberry Compote Granita

Ingredients

- 2 cups frozen blueberries
- 2 tablespoons lemon juice
- 2 tablespoons sugar
- 3 tablespoons water
- ½ cup cold water
- ¼ teaspoons freshly grated ginger (optional)

Directions

Prepare the compote as outlined here. Puree the compote, water and ginger until smooth. Taste for desired sweetness.

Pour the blueberry mixture into a 9- x 9- x 2-inch glass baking pan and put into the freezer. After 30 minutes, with a fork scrape the icy pieces. Every 30 minutes continue to scrape until you have a flaky light texture. Serve or keep in an airtight container in the freezer, scraping every so often to keep a light texture.

27. Cucumber Granita

Ingredients

- 3 cups cucumber, peeled and diced
- ½ cup cold water
- 2 limes, zested and juiced
- Pinch salt
- 2 tablespoons sugar
- 6 mint leaves

Directions

1. Puree all ingredients until smooth. Taste for sweetness.
2. Pour the cucumber juice into a 9 x 9 x 2-inch glass baking pan and put into the freezer. After 30 minutes, with a fork scrape to form flaky texture. Continue to scrape the surface every 30 minutes until you have a fluffy snowy consistency. Serve or keep in an airtight container in the freezer, scraping every so often to keep a light texture.

28. Green Tea Granita

Ingredients

- 2 green tea bags
- 1 cup hot water
- 1 tablespoon granulated sugar

Directions

Steep the green tea bags in hot water for 10 minutes. Discard bags.

Stir in the sugar and pour the mixture into a 9 by 9 inch baking pan. Cover and put into the freezer.

After 1 hour, using a fork, scrape the frozen top layer. Scrape and break frozen blocks into pieces. Continue to scrape every 15 to 20 minutes until the granita has a fluffy, snowy consistency – about 2 hours. Eat immediately or keep for 3 days, scraping every so often.

29. Grapefruit Granita

Ingredients

- 2 medium grapefruits
- 2 to 3 tablespoons agave

Directions

1. Roll the grapefruit on the countertop, pressing down on the fruit with the palm of your hand. This will loosen the rind and pith from the fruit.

2. Cut the tops and the bottoms off the grapefruit. Stand upright and cut downward around the shape of the grapefruit to remove the rind and pith.

3. To cut out the segments: over a bowl, take a paring knife and cut into the center of the fruit along each side of the white membrane that separates each segment. Gently pull the segments out and drop them into the bowl along with any resulting juice.

4. Using a stand blender or immersion blender, puree the grapefruit segments and juice with the agave. Taste for sweetness.

5. Pour into a 9- by 9-inch baking pan. Cover and put into the freezer.

6. After 1 hour, using a fork, scrape the frozen top layer. Scrape and break the frozen blocks into pieces. Continue to scrape every 15 to 20 minutes until the granita has a fluffy, snowy consistency – about 2 hours. Eat immediately or keep for 3 days, scraping every so often.

30. Lemon Ginger Granita

Ingredients

- 2 inch piece of fresh ginger, peeled and grated
- ½ cup water
- ¼ cup fresh lemon juice
- 3 tablespoons granulated sugar

Directions

1. Stir the ginger, water and lemon juice together. Stir in the sugar and pour the mixture into a 9- by 9-inch baking pan. Cover and put into the freezer.

2. After 1 hour, using a fork, scrape the frozen top layer. Scrape and break frozen blocks into pieces. Continue to scrape every 15 to 20 minutes until the granita has a fluffy, snow consistency, about 2 hours. Eat immediately or keep for 3 days in the freezer, scraping every so often.

Made in the USA
Monee, IL
21 August 2024